"Black Jack" To Get Your Health Back

A guide to wellness and to feel
and look great forever!

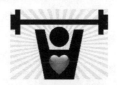

Carpe Diem

Seize the day—every day!

Stacey Karseras, LPN

authorHOUSE®

AuthorHouse™
1663 Liberty Drive
Bloomington, IN 47403
www.authorhouse.com
Phone: 1-800-839-8640

www.blackjacktolosefat.info

Published by AuthorHouse 4/17/12

ISBN: 978-1-4685-7221-6 (sc)
ISBN: 978-1-4685-7220-9 (hc)
ISBN: 978-1-4685-7222-3 (e)

Library of Congress Control Number: 2012906974

This book is printed on acid-free paper.

Credits

Concorde Career Institute CNA
The School of Fitness and Nutrition Phoenix, AZ certification in fitness and nutrition
Erwin Technical Center School of Nursing LPN

Contents

PREFACE

At the age of four, I asked my grandfather what the odd-shaped thing was at the foot of his bed. He told me it was a dumbbell (or free weight) that he used frequently to stay strong and healthy. My grandfather survived WWII and health problems because he has always remained fit and alert. His mind is still sharp; he lives alone and he will soon celebrate his ninety-second birthday. I always enjoy his history lessons and stories about his past. I dedicate this book to him.

Growing up, I didn't realize the impact that this type of lifestyle would provide long term, but it is never too late to become active, healthy, and fit. I spent most of my life at home and missed out on a good part of my life because I did not feel well. I obtained better health with the information I provide in *"Black Jack" To Lose Fat* and *"Black Jack" to Get Your Health Back*. With over twenty-five years of experience in healthcare, and through the eighteen thousand patients with whom I've completed pre-op interviews in just the last five years, I learned that many people are uneducated about their own health and do not know how to get their health back.

I have observed firsthand what repercussions poor health has on people's bodies—including my own—and I did not want to become a patient, so I developed a program that I have been able to commit to for thirty minutes, three days a week, in the comfort of my own home. In less than two years I have been able to decrease my body fat percentage, my measurements, and my size. I feel and look better than ever, and I no longer miss out on life.

Look for *"Black Jack" To Prevent a Surgery Setback* and use the three handbooks to remain healthy and fit or reclaim your life back forever. Carpe diem—seize the day!

INTRODUCTION

My first book "Black Jack" To Lose Fat was dedicated to my father. Many times, I listened to him after a visit to one of his physicians. He was sad, afraid, and disappointed with himself because he did not know how to get his health back. Once a healthy man, he became unfit due to lifestyle and habits. He tried several diets and diet gimmicks without long-term success, and his lifestyle and habits caught up with him. He had to have several surgeries; in addition, he consumed a lot of medication just to stay alive, and this pattern took a toll on his overall health and well-being.

The human body is built to perform, and the performance is both voluntary and involuntary because several organ systems work together to keep us alive and each one relies on the others for support. If one or more systems are compromised, the body does not function properly, and this determines our health.

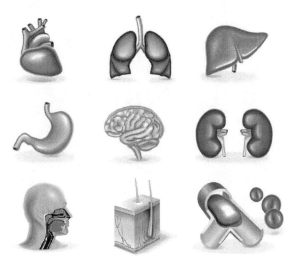

Our lifestyle and habits may affect the organs or cause illness and health problems. During our childhood, we tend to follow the lead of our caregivers and begin to model their behaviors. As we get older and begin to make our own decisions, we become our own caregivers or personal trainers. Something can be considered a habit if the action is repeated regularly for more than three weeks. The decision to look younger from head to toe begins with consistent resistance training and proper nutrition that becomes a lifestyle.

Growing up, I was not a picky eater but was always hungry and often felt nauseous, especially in the morning! I experienced IBS (irritable bowel syndrome), joint pain, chronic headaches, nausea, and vomiting. As I reached puberty, I began to experience PMS (premenstrual syndrome), mood swings, debilitating cramps every month, anxiety, and depression. I was exhausted all the time and did not sleep well. I tried to take medications and supplements for relief, but these products made me sicker. Over time, my own lifestyle and habits caught up with me. As my body fat percentage steadily increased, I experienced other health problems, such as borderline hypertension, elevated cholesterol, acid reflux, sleep apnea, and chronic sinusitis. For almost three years, I couldn't smell or taste and finally decided to have sinus surgery, but afterward I still experienced the same symptoms. I felt like a hypochondriac and was sick of being sick! Most of my life, I missed days from school, work, or functions with family and friends because I did not feel well. I even missed my own graduation from nursing school because of a headache and vomiting.

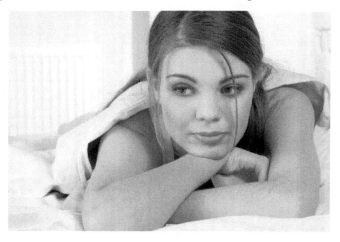

For a long time, I did not fully understand the adverse effects that improper nourishment and lack of resistance training have on the body, both physically and mentally. The body responds to activity and everything we consume whether it is food, beverages, prescribed medications, supplements, nicotine, alcohol, or recreational/illegal drugs. All of these things affect an individual's health, mood, behavior, inflammation or pain levels, and productivity. What we consume every day will determine the way we look and feel. I was a fan of dining out, fast food, and soda, and I had to gradually decrease how often I indulged in those things; so I began to prepare most of my meals and changed my lifestyle and habits. In two months I decreased my soda consumption from six liters a week to a shot glass, and today I no longer keep soda in the house. Every once in a while I will drink a soda, and I cannot believe how sweet it tastes and the amount of sugar it contains.

When I began to fuel my body frequently with proper nutrition and performed resistance training consistently, my health problems gradually diminished, including my chronic headaches and sinusitis. Almost every day, I pack my backpack/cooler with plenty of food and water to fuel my body and provide myself with energy throughout the day.

I developed a program that includes proper nutrition that tastes great and a resistance training program called "Black Jack" 21 that is included in my book *"Black Jack" To Lose Fat*. "Black Jack" 21 shapes the whole body in one circuit, and I recommend people complete the routine three days a week for optimum health benefits. In the summer of 2010, I began the journey to better health, and in less than two years I changed my life. I no longer have health problems or miss time with my family, friends, or work because I do not feel well. Since I have decreased my percentage of body fat, my size, and my measurements, I feel stronger and more alive. I feel better than ever and notice changes every week. Others tell me I look ten years younger than my age, and it feels good to feel good along with the added benefit of looking good. Jane Fonda and Richard Simmons have used resistance training and proper nutrition to sculpt their fabulous physiques for most of their lives—and what great energy and spirit they both project!

Everything we consume has an inflammatory response and can cause inflammation anywhere in the body, resulting in histamine reactions such as sinus congestion and skin problems. Sometimes, inflammation is caused by an environmental or seasonal type of allergen, but more often the problem is related to something we consume. There are many food products that have the same inflammatory response as many plant pollens, and the easiest way to find out what causes these reactions (besides being poked over one hundred times with a needle by an allergist) is to make a daily diary of your intake, health issues, environmental factors, and so forth. After a period of time, you may be able to pinpoint a few causes, especially if reactions occur after you consume dairy, nuts, wheat, or gluten products. I made a health diary for four years and learned a lot from my own body. I learned that I experienced sinus congestion and other symptoms with the fluctuation of hormones such as estrogen every month; smoking, exposure to smoke, air conditioning or heat; and some food and beverage items. Sometimes, using certain hair accessories or experiencing eye strain caused headaches. As long as I avoid these triggers, fuel my body properly, and perform "Black Jack" 21 three times a week I do not experience any health problems or symptoms.

Always seek medical advice prior to beginning any fitness or nutritional program.

DEFINITIONS

Affect: A person's mood or emotion

Antibiotics: A drug classification for medicine used to kill bacteria (not viruses, which cause illnesses such as the flu or common cold)

Antibiotic resistance: This occurs if antibiotics are taken over a period of time for conditions other than bacterial infections, causing a person to become resistant

Arteriosclerosis: A loss of elasticity in the walls of the arteries due to thickening and hardening from plaque, which impairs the circulation of the blood

Arthrosclerosis: A progressive process caused by the accumulation of plaque on the walls of the arteries

Aura: A personal radiance or glow

Bacterium: A microorganism of good or bad bacteria

Blood vessels: Arteries, veins, and capillaries that transport oxygenated blood and other substances throughout the body

Carotenoids: The red, yellow, orange, or dark green pigments found in fresh fruits and vegetables

Capillary: The webbed network between the arteries and veins where the interchange of oxygen, carbon dioxide, and nutrients take place

Cathartics: A product that assists with the motility of a bowel movement or defecation

Centurion: A person that lives to be one hundred years of age or older

Circulatory system: The system that promotes blood motility throughout the body via arteries, capillaries, and veins

Cirrhosis: A formation of fibrous tissue, scarring, and nodules that interfere with liver function and blood circulation

Defecation: The voluntary ability to expel a bowel movement or empty the rectum of feces or waste

Effect: A response or result

Endorphins: Neurotransmitters that aid in regulating the heart, hormone function, and the perception of pain, emotions, and motivation

Enriched flour: Flour that has been stripped of its natural nutrients and replaced with artificial nutrients, chemicals, and additives to prolong shelf life

Fever: A temperature above normal

Fibrosis: The scarring of fibrous tissue caused by irritation, inflammation, and healing

Flavonoids: Compounds (found in food or beverages) that contain antioxidants that decrease free radicals

Fortified: A product that has additives, such as vitamins and minerals (e.g., fortified cereal)

Free Radicals: Many of these agents may cause health problems or disease and are present in the environment

Gluten: A protein found in products processed with wheat, rye, or barley and adds the chewy texture to many baked goods

Legumes: A pod that splits on each side (e.g., peanuts, soybeans, peas, and beans)

Liver: An organ that receives and processes chemical substances in the blood according to the needs of the body

LRSA/Linezolid-Resistant *Staphylococcus Aureus*: A bacterial infection resistant to Linezolid antibiotics

MRSA/Methicilin-Resistant *Staphylococcus Aureus*: A bacterial infection resistant to Methicilin antibiotics

Preservatives: Additives, stabilizers, fillers, binders, flavor enhancers, colors, or dyes that are added to a food or beverage product to prolong shelf life by means of processing, canning, freezing, salting, pickling, or smoking

Processed: Any food or beverage item that goes through a process to enhance its flavor, color, or shelf life

Respiration: The exchange of oxygen and carbon dioxide through inhaling and exhaling when taking breaths

Sepsis: A response by the body to a bacterial infection that has entered the blood and tissues

Septic shock: A response that may occur if a person becomes septic, which may include high or low temperature, low blood pressure, rapid heart beat or breathing, chills, shaking, confusion, and decreased urination

Stressor: An occurrence that may cause an emotional or physical change

Shelf life: The length of time a product can safely be consumed or sold

Urination: The ability to expel fluid and waste products through the urinary system to the outside of the body

Virus: A microorganism that invades the body and can cause a viral infection (e.g., strains of the flu or common cold)

Wheat: A grain that is included in many food products and may cause allergies or other health problems

HEALTH PROBLEMS

Many circumstances determine our health, and sometimes we cause our own health problems due to lifestyle, habits, and activity level. A family history may predispose a person to a health problem, but almost everyone can prevent health problems with consistent resistance training and proper nutrition. Sometimes, family history means that other family members have lived a lifestyle that caused health problems, but unless you inherited a condition genetically or were born with a congenital problem, this history can be reversed. As previously mentioned, we model the behavior observed from our caregivers, and it is up to us to gain control of our lifestyles, take responsibility, be accountable for our own actions, and educate ourselves because once a health problem develops, the issue is much more difficult to diagnose or treat.

Treatments, medications, supplements, and food or beverage items may exacerbate symptoms because the side effects, adverse reactions, and allergies can cause secondary health problems. The body reacts differently to foreign objects, and these reactions may cause inflammation, infection, illness, disease, and cancer. Anyone who takes medications or supplements should be cautious, especially if taking more than one at a time or different kinds at the same time, due to the possibility of drug interactions. Many medications are used inappropriately or for recreational use, which can cause unpleasant outcomes and even death. These products are manufactured and include chemicals, preservatives, additives, and dyes with unknown short- and long-term effects.

Many times, a patient is looking for a quick fix to a problem and instead of changing his or her lifestyle or habits, and the person will consume numerous medications and supplements, or have surgery.

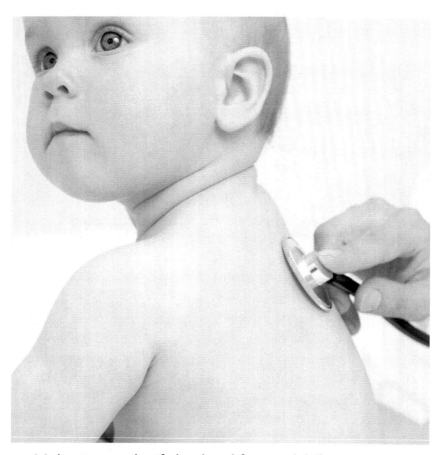

Medications are classified and used for several different reasons (such as antibiotics for bacterial infections); but these medications are becoming less effective, and usually a bacterium should be cultured to determine proper treatment. Unnecessary exposure to antibiotics may compromise a person and make it more difficult to treat an individual who requires an antibiotic to kill a bacterium in the future. Certain strains of *Staphylococcus aureus* infections (such as LRSA and MRSA) are resistant to antibiotics. MRSA used to be a hospital-acquired infection because it is easily spread through contact by healthcare employees. Hand washing continues to be the best defense for prevention or transmission of this bacterium.

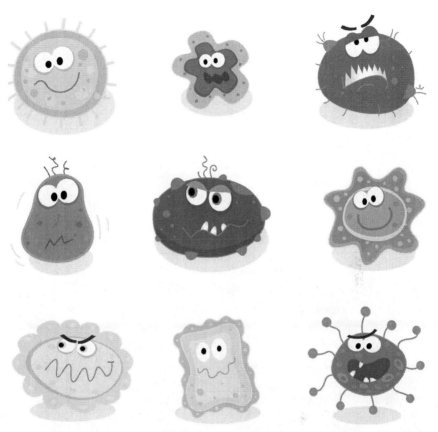

Anyone who has a weakened immune system for any reason may have a difficult time preventing or killing these or other strains of bacterium even with the proper medication or treatment. Good and bad bacteria such as MRSA lie dormant in and on our body at all times and can become active if contact is made with the live bacterium. Bacteria are easily picked up by direct contact, such as sharing towels, wash cloths or sponges, razors, exercise mats, and indoor or outdoor gym equipment. And, even beach sand has proven to be a host. Bug or dog bites, pimples, wounds, ingrown hairs or boils, burns, cellulites, abscesses, and sites where tubing enters the skin are all susceptible to this live bacterium. This bacterium can invade the skin, urine, bone, heart, eyes, and blood; and if MRSA infects the blood, sepsis and death can occur, so it is very important to treat a wound immediately and monitor the wound appropriately to prevent an infection from entering other areas of the body.

THE EFFECTS THAT NOURISHMENT HAS ON THE BODY

Certain types of nourishment can be unknowingly toxic, sabotage a person's health, and cause serious allergic reactions or health problems, such as obesity; hypertension; unstable metabolism, hormones, thyroid, or blood sugar levels; skin conditions; sinus congestion; cirrhosis of the liver; and elevated cholesterol levels, including triglycerides.

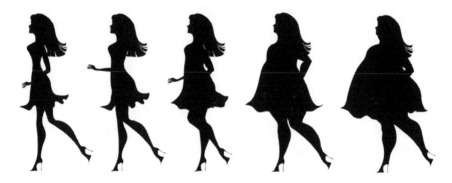

Obesity has become a worldwide epidemic, and statistics show that foreign countries now have an increased amount of health problems since the fast-food industry has occupied their cities. People are stretching their stomachs, consuming too much food too fast, making poor choices, eating simple carbohydrates full of starch and sugar, and waiting until hunger pangs are present before eating. Learn to walk away from a meal or snack without feeling full to prevent gastrointestinal discomfort. Everyone should try and avoid the all-you-can-eat establishments because of the urge to overeat and the increased risk of contracting viral or bacterial infections.

A healthy man named Morgan Spurlock decided to film a documentary called super size me while consuming fast food for thirty days. He consumed three meals a day at the same establishment, and his rule was that every time he was asked to supersize his meal he had to accept. His activity included walking a minimum of five thousand steps per day (or two and a half miles).

On day one, he weighed 185.5 pounds and had 11 percent body fat. After a couple of days, he experienced the sweats, nausea and vomiting, gas, bloating, and muscle twitching. Shortly after a meal, he was hungry again and craved more of the food.

Three supersized meals at a fast-food restaurant can contain as much as a pound or 453.6 grams of sugar. A twelve-ounce can of coke equals 39 grams of sugar per serving, and the average size soda is twenty-four ounces. The RDA or recommended daily allowance of sugar is only 40 grams per day!

After five days, the man had gained ten pounds. He felt depressed for no reason and experienced chest pain for the first time in his life. A team of physicians who monitored his health during this time recommended he abort the study because of the increased sodium intake, hypertension, (high blood pressure) headaches, body aches, and the fact that his liver was turning to fat.

After twelve days, he had gained seventeen pounds. After thirty days, he had gained 24.5 pounds; his liver did turn to fat; his cholesterol increased sixty five points; and his body fat increased to 18 percent. He doubled his risk for heart disease, and he felt short of breath after climbing one flight of stairs.

Most chicken nuggets are made from chickens that are fed hormones; nuggets contain additives, fillers, and preservatives to prolong shelf life. A chicken salad with a packet of ranch dressing is equivalent to a Big Mac; both contain approximately 51 grams of fat. A teacher conducted an experiment in which she placed a fast-food hamburger on her desk and left it untouched; thirty days later the hamburger remained the same (but hard as a rock) because of the preservatives.

The owners of two popular brands of ice cream also suffered with lifelong chronic health problems, and a person who drank a lot of diet soda temporarily lost his eyesight. Diet soda and sugar free products contain artificial sweeteners that may cause cancer in laboratory animals and predispose individuals to health problems, but we continue to place ourselves at risk by consuming these products. An unhealthy person may have chronic illness, disease, or cancer, and there aren't any benefits to consuming improper nourishment, too much food at one time, the same thing every day, or skipping meals. Avoiding fresh fruits, vegetables, and dairy products will cause health problems, including nutrient deficiencies, inflammation, mood swings, and unstable metabolism, hormones, thyroid, or blood sugar levels.

Americans are used to everything being big; a bigger bang for the buck always sounds better, and most fast-food chains have a dollar menu. These establishments have popped up on every corner, and some establishments include meals with toys and play areas for children. We are predisposing ourselves and our loved ones to health problems when we don't provide proper nutrition on a consistent basis. Since most people dine out the majority of the time, fresh home-cooked meals have become a thing of the past.

It is important for better health to consume natural, fresh, or frozen items and to combine all the food groups at the right time for a healthy balance. Eat lean proteins, complex carbohydrates, and healthy fats together every three to four hours while awake, and avoid consuming meals or beverages two hours prior to falling asleep.

THE HEART

A healthy adult heart is approximately nine to eleven ounces. It has four chambers and is a muscular pump that contracts rhythmically, circulating blood to the lungs and the body through arteries and valves. An unhealthy heart can become enlarged and cause health problems such as unstable blood pressure or heart rate.

The organs in the body respond to high blood pressure, and if left untreated, chances of a heart attack, stroke, arteriosclerosis, kidney damage, poor eyesight, and other health problems increase.

To decrease the risks, a few simple changes can be made, such as consuming less processed convenience food, alcohol, and nicotine. Drinking more water, eating fresh or frozen fruits and vegetables, natural products, and products with low glycemic index values or inflammatory responses helps a great deal as well—as does adding a resistance training program like "Black Jack" 21 or "Black Jack" 21 the advanced version to strengthen the cardiovascular system and increase health benefits.

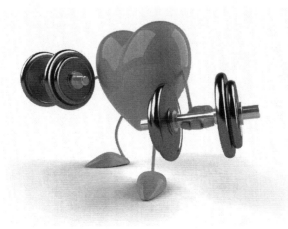

Two important components for heart health are vitamin K for clotting purposes and potassium for proper cell, tissue, and organ function. Sometimes, potassium is removed from the body due to health problems and medications. Decreased potassium is also linked to leg and muscle cramps.

Unhealthy cholesterol including triglycerides can collect in the arteries causing improper blood flow, blockages, heart attack, or stroke, and may even break off from the wall of the artery creating a pulmonary embolus (blood clot) that can travel throughout the body; this is very dangerous and can result in death. Annual check-ups and frequent blood lab draws are usually performed on patients who have health problems.

The Lungs

Most of us are born with two lungs, which are located inside the diaphragm in front of the chest wall. These organs are responsible for air exchange as we inhale and exhale. While we sleep, the action is involuntary, and while we are awake, it becomes voluntary due to skeletal muscle contraction.

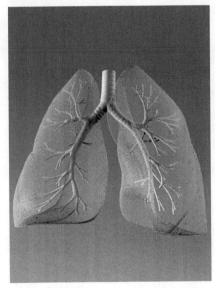

Many factors can decrease our lung function including health problems, illness, environmental or seasonal conditions, smoking, and smoke. Once lung damage is present, it cannot be reversed, but overall lung function, oxygen saturation, and energy levels can improve greatly over time.

Resistance training is an anaerobic activity and aids in increased lung function due to the increased oxygen levels produced in the blood during this type of exercise.

THE URINARY SYSTEM

Most of us are born with two kidneys, and their primary function is to remove waste from the blood through urination, produce a hormone that aids in the formation of red cells, and stabilize salts and other substances in the blood.

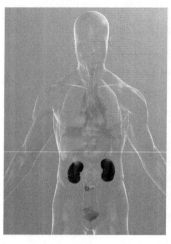

Two narrow tubes called ureters carry urine from the kidneys to the bladder. The bladder stores the urine, which is propelled by the contraction of the sphincter muscles through the urethra to the outside of the body during urination.

This natural process can be compromised due to health problems, illness, bladder weakness, or injury to the spinal cord or pelvic floor. Other causes may be medications, diuretics, spinal cord injuries, surgeries, and the aging process. Food and beverage products can also alter urinary health including the color, scent, and volume of urine. Urine should be a slight yellow color but almost clear and should not smell bad. Secondary conditions and food products that are processed or that contain sodium may increase one's urine output and potentially cause edema or water retention throughout the body as well as high blood pressure, which causes the kidneys to work harder.

Kegel exercises can be performed by females and males to strengthen the muscle that allows one to hold urine and to decrease weakness and frequency of urination, which will help prevent leakage or incontinence.

Neurological Problems

The central nervous system includes the brain and the spinal cord. The brain controls the organ systems and instructs the body to perform, feel, remember, and imagine. The brain stem contains organs that regulate hormones and body processes. The items we consume daily and our level of fitness will determine the secretion or stability. The spinal cord permits an active range of motion, motor and sensory impulses, urination, and defecation. Messages are carried by neurons to keep the body functioning properly.

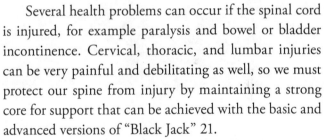

Several health problems can occur if the spinal cord is injured, for example paralysis and bowel or bladder incontinence. Cervical, thoracic, and lumbar injuries can be very painful and debilitating as well, so we must protect our spine from injury by maintaining a strong core for support that can be achieved with the basic and advanced versions of "Black Jack" 21.

Headaches can also be debilitating, and determining the cause, trigger, or treatment can be frustrating. Triggers can include hunger, dehydration, alcoholic or other beverages, food products, medications, supplements, environmental or seasonal elements, smoking or smoke, and hair accessories. Products that are processed, red wine (which contains sulfites and tannins), chocolate, hot dogs (which contain nitrates), and ice cream are all common triggers, and by process of elimination some headaches and other health problems may be avoided.

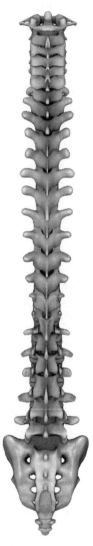

Numbness and tingling in the extremities are two other problems that can be serious or a secondary condition due to other health problems or medications including supplements, but these sometimes occur while one is asleep because of body positioning. If extremities such as the ankles, legs, arms, or hands are folded, crossed, or clenched for example: the fetal position circulation may become compromised. Simple changes, repositioning the body, and using pillows for support may prevent unnecessary symptoms.

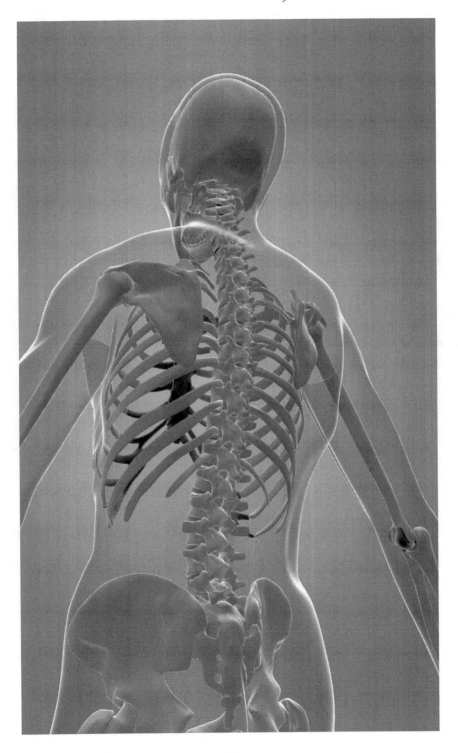

The Digestive Tract

Anything a person consumes travels from his or her mouth down the esophagus to the stomach through the colon and intestines and is then expelled through the rectum to the outside of the body. If this does not occur naturally, then other measures may have to be taken to promote defecation. Health problems, sedentary lifestyles, and intestinal or spinal cord injuries place people at risk for bowel problems. Pain medications increase the risk for constipation, and antibiotics increase the risk for gastrointestinal discomfort and diarrhea.

Food should be flushed with plenty of water; this is particularly true when it comes to processed food items since they contain extra sodium/salt and by-products. Nourishment choices, medications, supplements, excessive vomiting, alcohol, excess weight, and smoking can cause irritation to the lining of the esophagus, stomach, and intestines. Chewing gum, drinking from a straw, or talking while eating can cause additional gas or bloating in the intestinal tract.

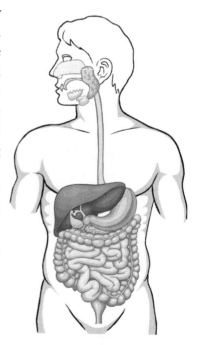

Gastrointestinal problems such as bloating, gas, indigestion, or acid reflux are other problems that may be prevented with consistent resistance training, proper nutrition, awareness, and prevention.

NOURISHMENT CHOICES THAT FUEL THE BODY

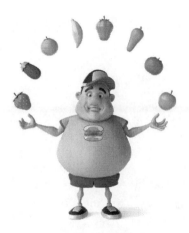

The nourishment choices we make affect the way we feel and behave everyday. Many choices can provide health benefits, increase energy levels and productivity, and decrease pain. Great examples of proper nutrition are fresh or frozen fruits and vegetables including apples, avocados, bananas, berries, cherries, citrus fruits, prunes, asparagus, broccoli, spinach, and other products such as spices, dairy products, fish, shrimp, poultry, lean red meat, legumes, nuts, seeds, and more healthy fats. These choices are high in vitamins, minerals, and flavonoids.

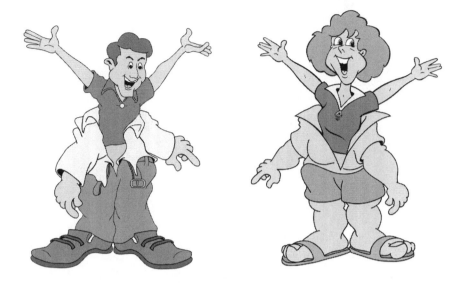

Products that contain mostly starch or sugar usually have higher glycemic index values, which spike blood sugar levels quickly and deplete energy, creating mood swings, inflammation, increased pain, low productivity, and decreased libido.

To receive an equal balance, consume protein, complex carbohydrates, and healthy fat together every three to four hours while awake. Try to avoid consuming meals or beverages two hours prior to sleeping.

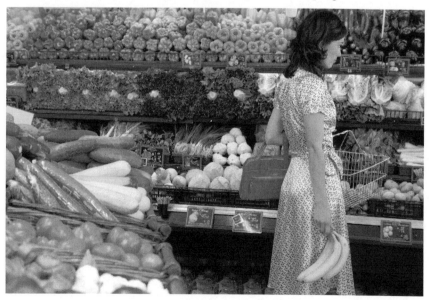

FLAVONOIDS

Flavonoids have antioxidant effects and may increase health benefits and boost the immune system. These compounds include phenols, tannins (contained in most wine), lycopene, quercetin, epicatechin, hesperidin, rutin, luteolin, apigenin, plant-named derivatives, vitamin P (P for pigment), and astaxanthin (a pigment responsible for the color of crustaceans). These compounds are responsible for providing color to most fruits and vegetables, which is the key to a high nutrient value. Some fruits and vegetables will lose nutrient values if refrigerated or not stored properly.

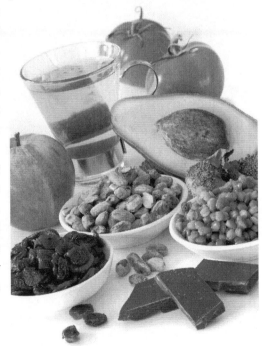

Dark chocolate, darker beans and red wine are also categorized as flavonoids. These compounds are found in the products that we should try to consume daily to prevent health problems and help build immunity.

Examples of Daily Intake

For optimum benefits, pack your food in a cooler or backpack cooler with an icepack to keep items cold throughout the day or use a thermos to keep items hot. Pack extra food to prevent hunger, cravings, and bingeing, and be sure to consume meals and snacks *before* you feel hungry, as this will stabilize the metabolism, hormones, thyroid, and blood sugar levels.

Example 1

7:00 a.m.
coffee with hazelnut creamer and sugar
water

8:00 a.m.
two eggs (scrambled)
one banana
milk
water

11:00 a.m.
½ PB&J
one serving of fruit (orange, prunes, mango, or ½ avocado)
water

2:00 p.m.
mozzarella string cheese
one serving of fruit
water

5:00 p.m.

pita chips
hummus
water

8:00 p.m.
shrimp
broccoli
pasta
water

10:00 p.m.
sleep

Example 2

7:00 a.m.
coffee with hazelnut creamer and sugar
water

9:00 a.m.
smoothie/milkshake
water

11:30 a.m.
lettuce mix with tomato and homemade tuna fish salad
one serving of fruit
water

3:00 p.m.
one serving of fruit
cheese
crackers
water
(The cheese/crackers can be zapped in the microwave.)

6:30 p.m.
homemade pasta salad (see recipe)
water

8:30 p.m.
cookies
milk

10:30 p.m.
sleep

Example 3

9:00 a.m.
smoothie or milkshake
water

11:30 a.m.
grilled cheese sandwich
one serving of fruit
water

3:00 p.m.
cookies
milk
water

7:00 p.m.
dinner and a movie (cinebistro)
blue crab sandwich and french fries w/ketchup
one or two favorite beverages
extra water

11:00 p.m.
sleep

Example 4

8:00 a.m.
three egg omelet w/cheese, peppers, mushrooms, and salsa
one serving of fruit
coffee with hazelnut creamer and sugar
water

12:00 p.m.
lunch out (chicken wrap)
water

2:00 p.m.

iced coffee or cappuccino
water

4:00 p.m.
apples
natural peanut butter
water

6:30 p.m.
curry chicken
jasmine rice
frozen spinach (thawed and cooked)
water

9:30 p.m.
frozen dark-chocolate-covered banana
milk

12:00 a.m.
sleep

Example 5

10:00 a.m.
cinnamon bun
two eggs
orange slices
milk

1:00 p.m.
coffee with creamer and sugar

4:00 p.m.
salsa
tortilla chips
water

6:30 p.m.
BBQ
coleslaw
pasta salad

bread
water

9:30 p.m.
sleep

Weekdays and weekends do not have to be a challenge anymore if you make healthier choices most of the time within moderation, and you can choose french fries or your favorite dessert just once in a while. Make the choices wisely, so you do not feel deprived.

It is important to eat frequently while awake to stabilize metabolism, hormones, thyroid, and blood sugar levels. Once you begin to fuel your body with proper nutrition and feel well, it is hard to revert back to the old lifestyle and habits. Something becomes a habit after three weeks, so gradually decrease the habits that are making you unhealthy and increase new habits to become healthy and fit for life. Do not try to cut anything cold turkey because the long-term success rate is very low.

RDA

The establishment of RDA (recommended daily allowances of nutrients) began in 1914 during WWI due to food rations and then became a guide for caloric intake, vitamins, and minerals. Allowances were made according to the nutritional values of the products available at that time due to the increased risk for health problems and vitamin or mineral deficiencies.

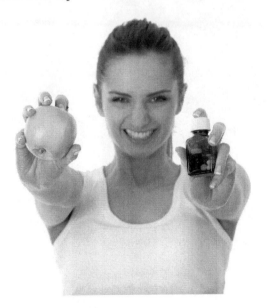

If nutrients are provided in the food we consume, than consuming additional nutrients (through vitamin and mineral supplements) isn't usually necessary and can actually cause harm and become toxic in the blood. Vitamins, minerals, and other supplements are not FDA approved and the benefits, if any, are not scientifically proven.

Caloric RDA

Carbohydrates	300 grams
Cholesterol	300 milligrams
Fat	65 grams
Fiber	25 grams
Potassium	4,700 milligrams
Protein	50 grams
Saturated Fat	20 grams
Sodium	2,300 milligrams
Sugar	40 grams

According to the Food and Nutrition Board the dietary reference intakes or DRI's are as follows: for males and females age nineteen to seventy. These are a few examples of foods with nutrient values

VITAMIN RDA

Vitamin A (Beta-Carotene) M (900 mcg) F (700 mcg)	carrots, spinach, sweet potato with skin, prunes, fortified cereal and peppers
Vitamin B1 (Thiamin) M (1.2 mg) F (1.1 mg)	whole grain/wheat products
Vitamin B2 (Riboflavin) M (1.3 mg) F (1.1 mg)	milk, fortified cereal, and fresh bread products
Vitamin B3 (Niacin) M (16 mg) F (14 mg)	fish, meat, poultry, fortified cereal, whole grain/wheat products, mushrooms, asparagus, and peanuts
Vitamin B5 (Pantothenic acid) M (5 mg) F (5 mg)	fortified cereal, chicken, beef, oats, potatoes, and tomatoes
Vitamin B6 (Pyridoxine) M (1.3–1.7 mg) F (1.3–1.5 mg)	fortified cereal, soy products, organ meats, whole grains, bran, chicken, eggs, garlic, and peppers
Vitamin B7 (Biotin) M (30 mcg) F (30 mcg)	fruits, liver, and meat

Vitamin B9 (Folate) M (400 mcg) F (400 mcg)	dark, leafy vegetables, whole grain/wheat products, and fortified cereal
Vitamin B complex (B1–B12)	eggs, liver, milk, and peanuts
Vitamin B12 (Cyanocobalmin) M (2.4 mcg) F (2.4 mcg)	fish, fortified cereal, meat, and poultry
Vitamin C (Ascorbic acid) M (90 mg) F (75 mg)	avocados, kiwi, citrus, peppers, strawberries, apples, peaches, pineapples, tomatoes, onions, broccoli, garlic, and peppers
Vitamin D (Calciferol) M (15–20 mcg) F (15–20 mcg)	fatty fish and fish oil, egg yolk, fortified cereal, yogurt, cheese, and milk
Vitamin D3 (Cholecalciferol) M (15mcg) F (15-20mcg)	exposure to natural sunlight and artificial sunlamps (ultraviolet irradiation)
Vitamin E (Alpha-tocopherol) M (15 mg) F (15 mg)	natural peanut butter, safflower oil, sunflower oil and olives and olive oil, almonds, hazelnuts, green, leafy vegetables, broccoli, blue crab, and rockfish, potatoes, avocados, tomatoes, and peppers
Vitamin K (Mephyton) M (120 mg) F (90 mg)	spinach, collards, broccoli, brussels sprouts, and avocadoes

MINERAL RDA

Calcium M (1,000 mg) F (1,000–1,200 mg)	milk, Greek yogurt, cheese, spinach, fortified cereal, and garlic
Chromium M (35–30 mg) F (25–20 mg)	fish, poultry, and meat
Copper M (900 mcg) F (900 mcg)	whole grain/wheat products, seeds, nuts, seafood, and prunes
Fluoride M (4 mg) F (3 mg)	fluoridated water and some seafood
Iodine M (150 mcg) F (150 mcg)	iodized salt and processed foods
Iron M (8 mg) F (8 mg)	beans, beef, and lentils
Manganese M (2.3 mg) F (1.8 mg)	beans, nuts, legumes, whole grain/wheat products, garlic, and peppers
Magnesium M (420 mg) F (320 mg)	almonds, Brazil nuts, soybeans, halibut, quinoa, and green, leafy vegetables

Molybdenum M (45 mcg) F (45 mcg)	grains, nuts, and legumes
Phosphorus M (700 mg) F (700 mg)	eggs, dairy products, milk, meat, peas, some cereal, bread products, and garlic
Potassium M (4.7 g) F (4.7 g)	bananas, prunes, Greek yogurt, yellow fin tuna, sweet potatoes, and soybeans
Selenium M (55 mcg) F (55 mcg)	Brazil nuts, organ meat, and seafood
Sodium (Sodium chloride) M (1.5–1.3 g) F (1.5–1.3 g)	salt, products with salt added, pickled, and processed items
Zinc M (11 mg) F (8 mg)	red meat, seafood, and fortified cereal

Inflammatory Response

Internal and external changes can occur inside and outside of the body. The inflammatory response can be a reaction to the products we consume, injuries, illness, or seasonal or environmental conditions. Proper prevention may alleviate allergens that release histamines and trigger inflammatory responses.

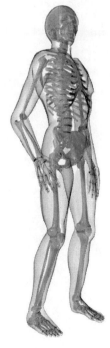

Food products such as spices, garlic, peppers, and other food products and beverages can be consumed to decrease inflammation. A great website that offers information on inflammation factors, glycemic index values, and nutritional data is nutritiondata.self.com.

Medications and Supplements

Medications and supplements are chemical compounds manufactured in factories; there are health risks involved in taking supplements, so take them at your own risk. Medications are regulated by the Food and Drug Administration, but supplements are not. Many medications are used to diagnose, treat, or prevent health problems. Medication trials and experiments are performed every day, and people experiment and receive compensation while consuming such products. Many times, the risk of taking a medication outweighs the benefits, and attorneys work with clients who experience poor outcomes. It is important to read the information included with any such products regarding possible adverse reactions, side effects, and allergies. Common side effects include headache, nausea, vomiting, constipation, and diarrhea, just to name a few; and allergic reactions can include unstable vital signs, rashes/hives, and even anaphylactic shock or swelling of the tongue and throat.

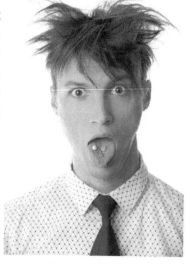

Medications and supplements have to be stored appropriately because air, light, heat, cold, and humidity alter the effects of these products. Some products cannot be taken together due to drug interactions. Medications should be taken according to the directions provided and the additional labeled information on the medication container. Medications should always be flushed with plenty of water, unless otherwise instructed, so as to prevent irritation to the lining of the esophagus and stomach.

The human immune system is built to resist and fight off foreign bodies. Often times, the body can defend itself, but if a person is immunocompromised, then it is more difficult to prevent an injury, infection, inflammation, illness, cancer, or gastrointestinal changes.

RECIPES AND "BLACK JACK" TIPS

Smoothies and Milk Shakes

These are considered high protein and include natural whey (from the Greek yogurt)

My typical 20-ounce drink includes:

2 cups of liquid

2 tbsp of vanilla yogurt

1 tbsp of peanut butter

1 cup fruit

½ tsp chocolate syrup

½ tsp cinnamon

Other variations are listed below the recipe.

Mix the ingredients listed below in a blender:

Ice (unless fruit is frozen)

Any type of milk or water

Greek yogurt (plain or vanilla)

Plain yogurt is not sweet if consumed by itself

Optional items include but aren't limited to natural peanut butter, cinnamon, dark chocolate syrup, coffee, cayenne pepper

Cayenne pepper speeds up the metabolism.

Fruit (any kind): blueberries, bananas, strawberries, peaches, mangos, etc.

"Black Jack" tip:
Most fruits can be frozen. For example, peel a banana and place it in a zipper-lock freezer bag. Most fruits can also be found already frozen. You should use the fruit within six months for optimum nutrient benefits.

Variations:
Coffee, milk, banana, natural peanut butter, cinnamon, and dark chocolate syrup
Banana and strawberry
Blueberry, banana, dark chocolate syrup, and natural peanut butter
Banana and natural peanut butter
Strawberry and blueberry
> **For an extra treat, line the inside of the cup with dark chocolate syrup and top your beverage with whipped cream**

Tuna or Egg Salad
Fresh cooked or canned tuna *or* chopped hardboiled eggs
Mayonnaise, Miracle Whip, or ranch or Italian dressing
Optional ingredients: mustard, onion, celery, tomatoes, sweet pickle relish, salt and pepper, curry powder
Mix ingredients and serve on bread, on a bed of lettuce, in a hollowed tomato or pepper, or mixed with cooked (chilled) pasta

Fresh Salsa
Diced tomatoes, onions, green peppers, fresh garlic and cilantro, salt and pepper
Mix together and serve with tortilla chips, with eggs, or mixed with cream cheese on crackers

"Black Jack" tip:
A dash of sugar will decrease the acid in the tomatoes

Pasta Salad

Chilled cooked pasta

Chilled cooked shrimp (peeled and deveined)

Optional ingredients: cucumbers, peppers, cherry or grape tomatoes

Mix together with Italian dressing

Serve cold

Curry Chicken

Cooked chicken

Coconut milk

Curry powder

Optional ingredients: rice, potatoes, broccoli, frozen, cut leaf spinach

BBQ

Beef, poultry, or fish

Barbecue sauce

A gas, electric, or charcoal grill

"Black Jack" tip:

For a smoked flavor just add flavored wood. Use a wood that will enhance the flavor of the food, for example, apple, blueberry, hickory, oak, pecan, mesquite, etc.

If you do not have a smoker or smoker box, then soak wood in water for a couple of hours and place wood directly over the coals.

"Black Jack" tip:

Direct or indirect heat may be used; slow cook the meat for hours.

Better Dining Choices

If dining out, it is easier to make better choices if small, more frequent meals and snacks are consumed throughout the day (every three to four hours). Choose an appetizer, share an entrée, or save the other half of your meal for later. If you have a career that requires traveling and dining out, making good choices will be a bit more challenging, but it can be accomplished. Try to balance your meal with protein, complex carbohydrates, and healthy fats, and incorporate fresh fruits with low glycemic index values three to four times daily with meals and snacks. Homemade, high-protein smoothies/milkshakes are a great balance and a delicious choice to provide energy. They are also a good way to consume a couple of servings of fruit, and they an excellent source of healthy whey protein.

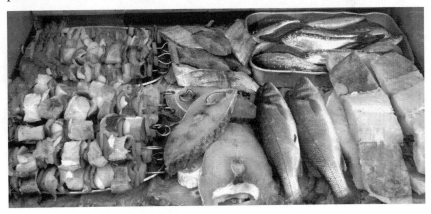

Be mindful of condiments, dressings, sauces, and soups (especially cream-based ones), as well as anything processed or enriched because these items can sabotage other health efforts. Soup may be filling and a healthy choice if it is homemade and made with milk (rather than cream) or clear broth. Canned soups contain too much sodium and are not recommended.

A salad can be satisfying if it contains fillers, such as meat, beans, legumes, or cheese. Foods high in starch should be avoided and should not be consumed by themselves due to the spike in blood sugar they cause, which is followed by a crash of energy. Fresh salsa can be added to eggs or grits, or mixed with cream cheese to make a delicious dip.

Choose items that will fuel the body, satisfy hunger between meals and snacks, and provide health benefits for the mind, body, and spirit throughout the day, every day.

The Muscles and Joints

Strong muscles and lubricated joints may support the body or prevent injury from occurring, but many injuries are caused by repetitive motion and too much weight bearing on a particular joint especially if the supporting muscle is already weak. Lack of mobility equals lack of motility, and the more sedentary you are, the weaker you will become. Resistance training goes back centuries. Hippocrates said, "That which is used develops, and that which is not, wastes." This type of training is proven to lower health risks, increase strength, stamina, and bone density, and provide other benefits as well. Anyone over the age 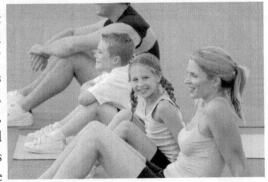 of four can use resistance to train. With proper supervision, the whole family can perform resistance exercises together such as the two programs I developed called "Black Jack" 21 and "Black Jack" 21 advanced version, three times a week. You'll develop a greater desire to gain strength and achieve the next hurdle in your life with greater ease.

Muscles that are strengthened by resistance continue to produce vitamins, minerals, and hormones naturally to increase energy; provide nutrients; and stabilize metabolism, hormone, thyroid, and blood sugar levels as well as blood pressure, mood, and pain levels. When you feel well and look good, others will want to know your secret

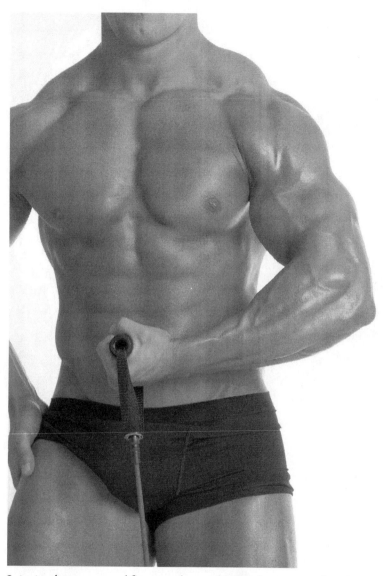

Injuries that are caused from weak muscles may be prevented with strength training, which increases lean muscle mass and tonicity to better support the joints. People who do not train with resistance and participate in sports for fun increase their risk of injuries because weak muscles cause weak joints.

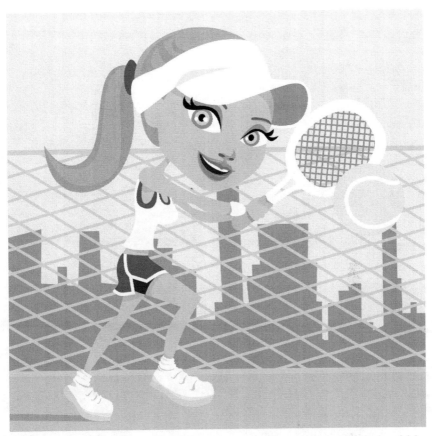

The motto "No pain, no gain" no longer applies, and the goal should be to eliminate pain, injury, and surgery.

ANATOMY OF THE HUMAN BODY

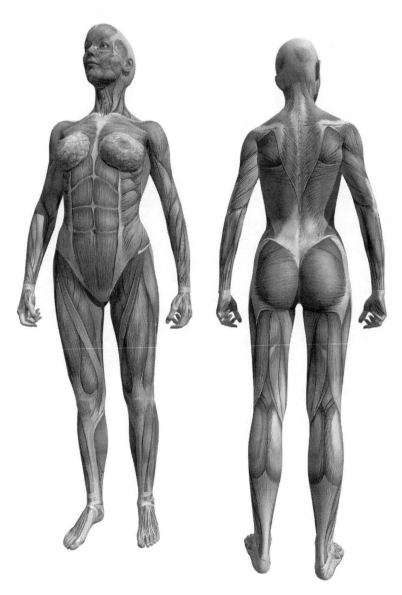

FEMALE

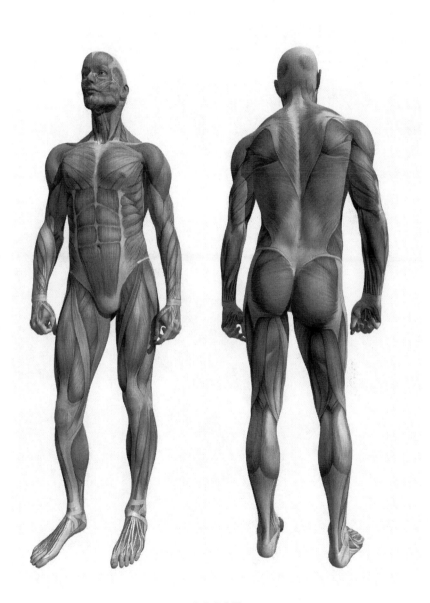

MALE

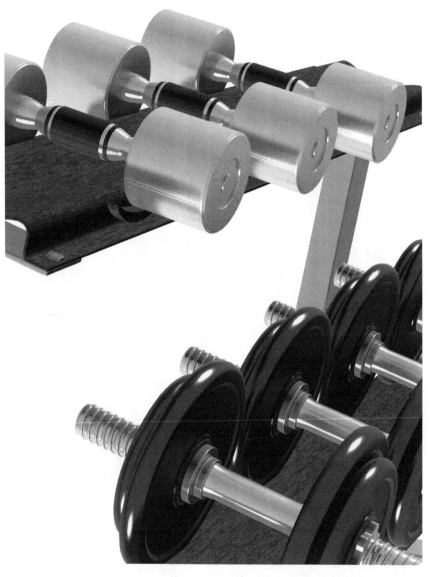

Resistance training can be achieved with just a dumbbell (free weight), a multi-station gym, or separate pieces of gym equipment. The least expensive and most versatile of these is the dumbbell workout. In addition, most exercises can be performed using both sides of the body at the same time or alternating each extremity.

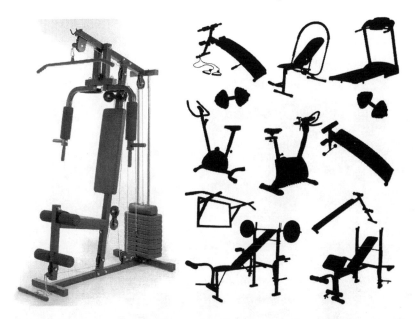

Each individual will have different capabilities depending on experience or strength. Start slowly and gradually making changes in your lifestyle for long-term success. Staying healthy and physically fit will require effort, but after a few months of consistent training, this lifestyle will become effortless because after each work out you become stronger.

This is the only program I have ever committed to because it takes approximately forty minutes three days a week. I can exercise in the comfort of my own space and listen to my favorite music. The health benefits and visual results also keep me coming back for more every week.

"BLACK JACK" 21: ADVANCED VERSION

Use the alternate "Black Jack" 21 and the advanced version to achieve better health. *The advanced version should not be performed more than three weeks in a row.* This is a great workout if you are preparing for a vacation or a special event.

Always warm up, cool down, and stretch
(before, during, and after a work out)

Perform each set and repeat. Using a different weight for each exercises as needed (the muscle should be slightly stressed towards the twelfth repetition of each exercise).

> fifteen concentration curls
> fifteen bicep curls
> fifteen hammer curls
>
> fifteen shoulder presses
> fifteen shoulder shrugs
> fifteen front raises
> fifteen bent-over lateral raises
>
> fifteen dead lifts
> fifteen squats
> fifteen calf raises

fifteen leg lifts
fifteen lunges

fifteen bent-over rows
fifteen tricep extensions
fifteen tricep kickbacks

Floor Routine

fifteen abdominal crunches
fifteen reversed abdominal crunches
fifteen flyes
fifteen leg lifts
fifteen leg curls
fifteen push ups

Concentration Curl

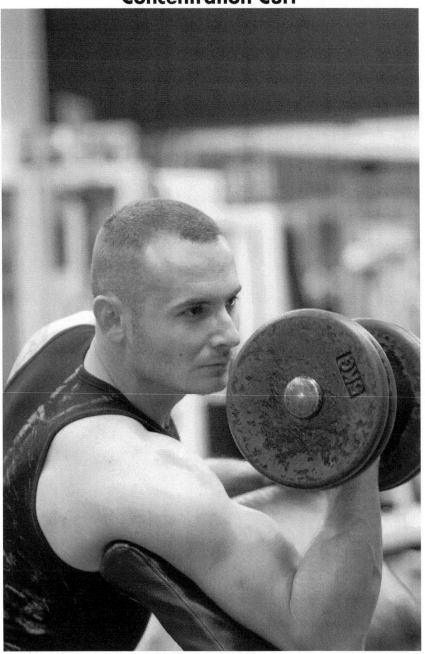

Concentration Curl

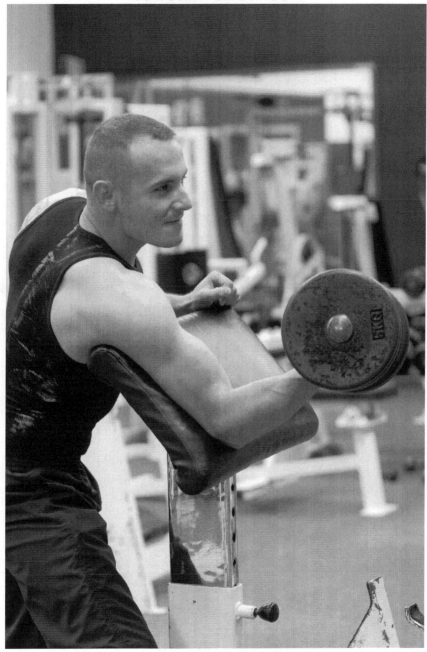

Bicep Curl

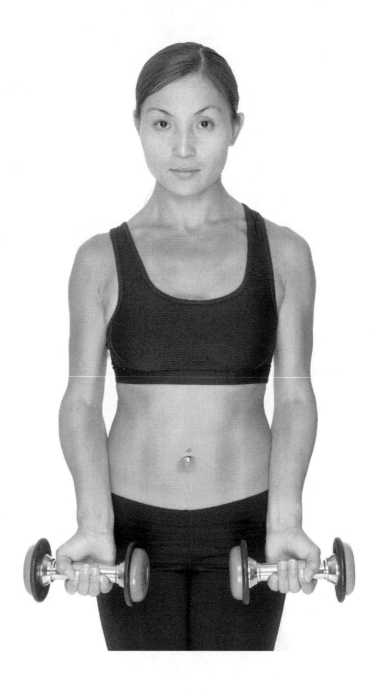

Bicep Curl

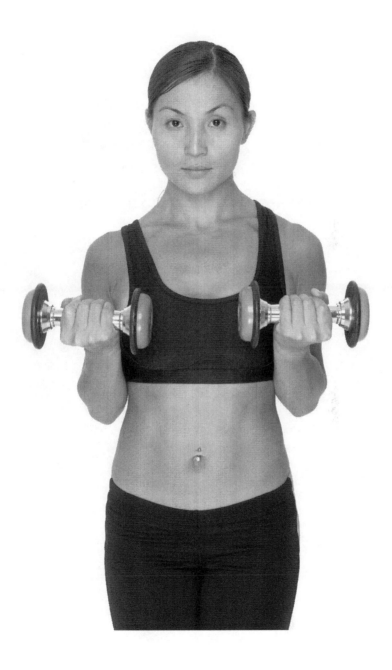

Hammer Curl

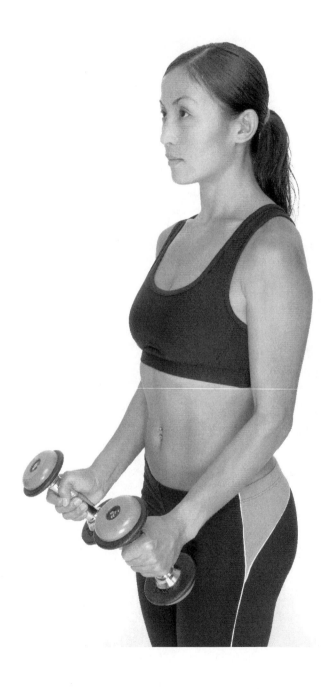

Hammer Curl

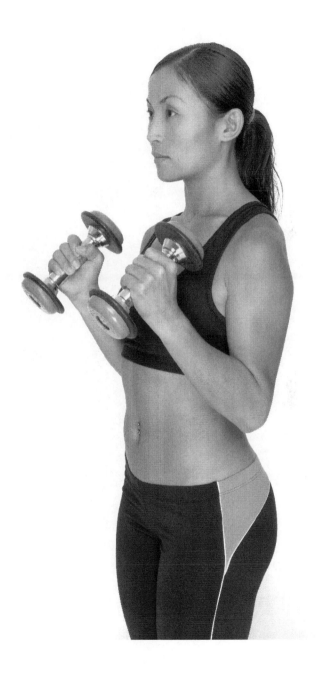

Shoulder Press

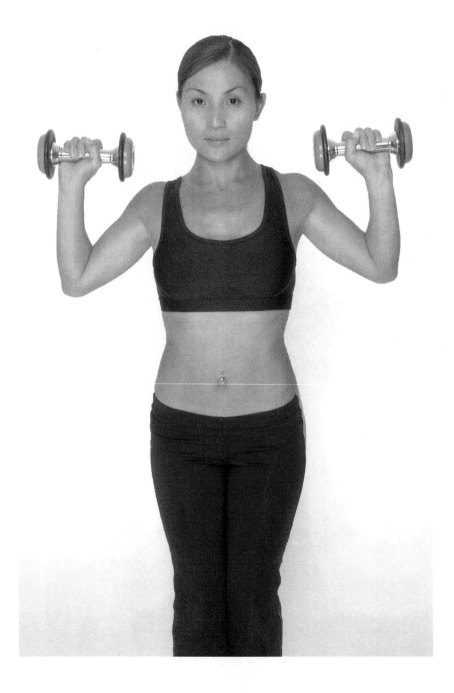

Shoulder Press

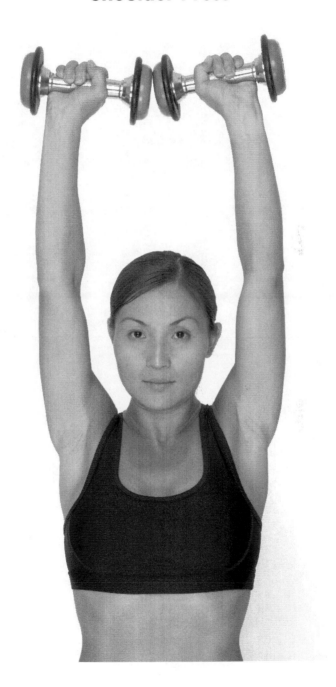

Shoulder Shrug

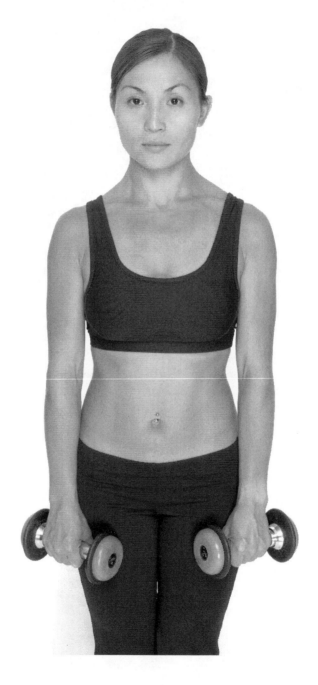

Shoulder Shrug

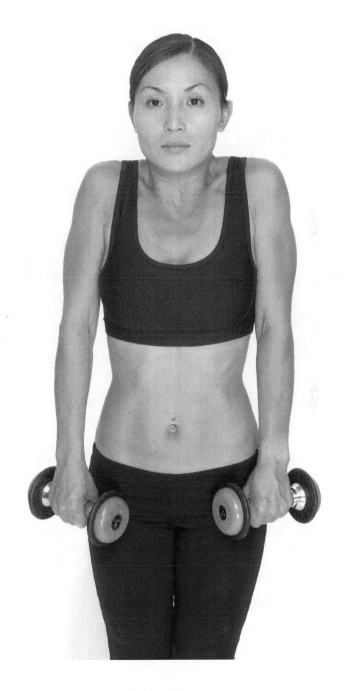

Front Raise

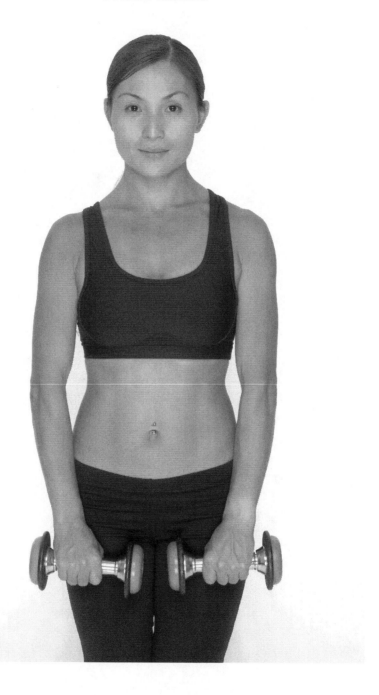

Front Raise

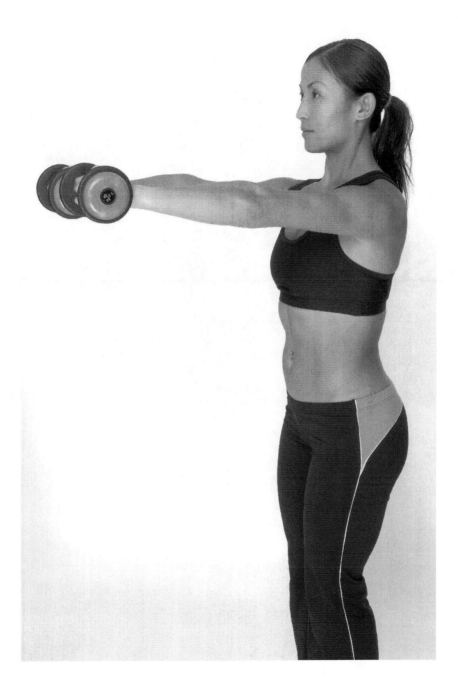

Bent-Over Lateral Raise

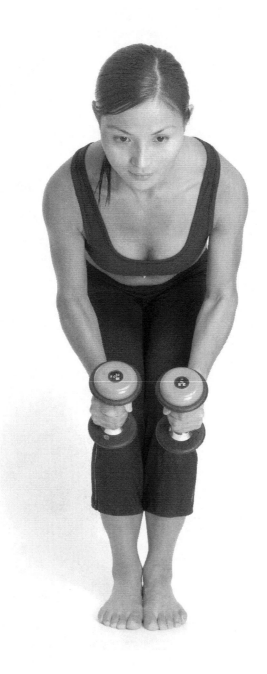

Bent-Over Lateral Raise

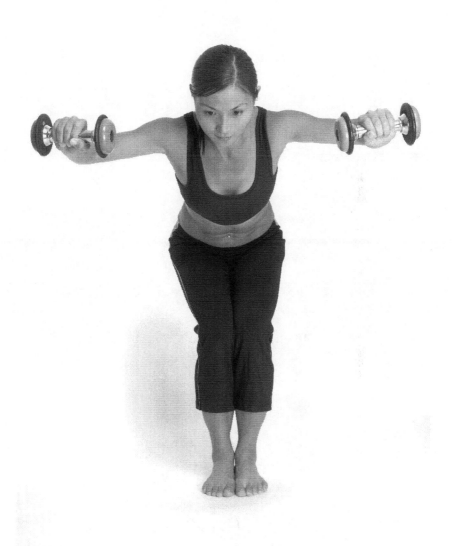

Dead Lift

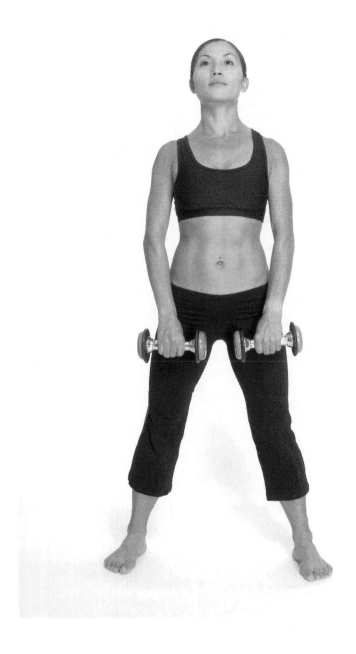

Dead Lift

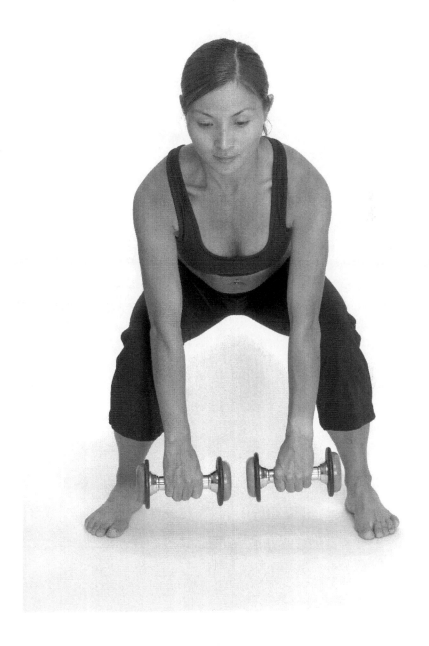

Squat

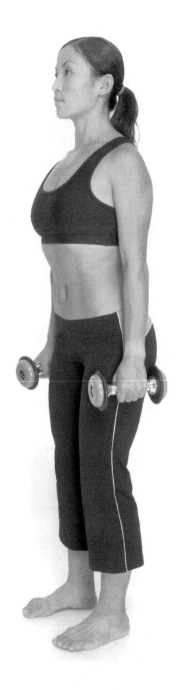

Squat

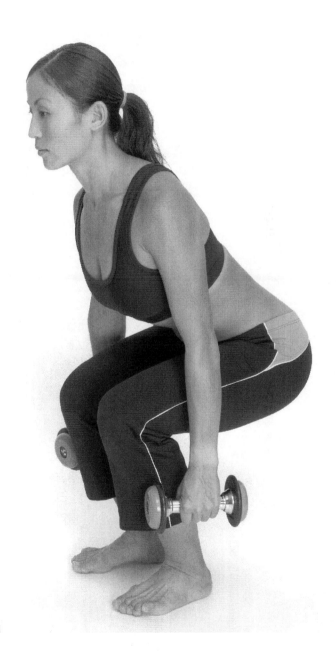

Calf Raise

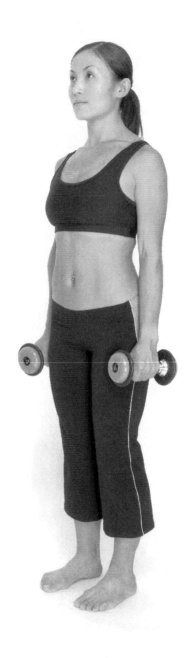

Calf Raise

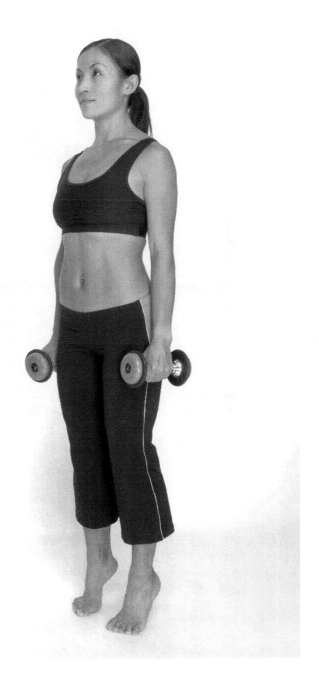

Leg Lift

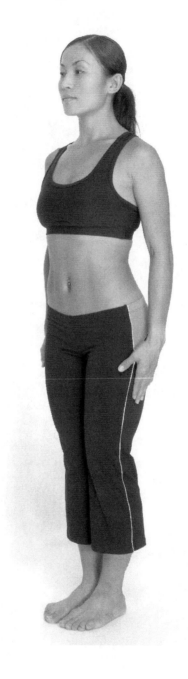

Leg Lift

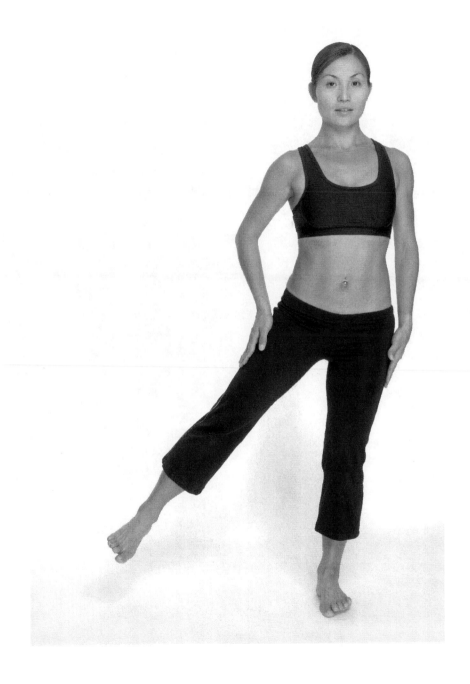

Lunge

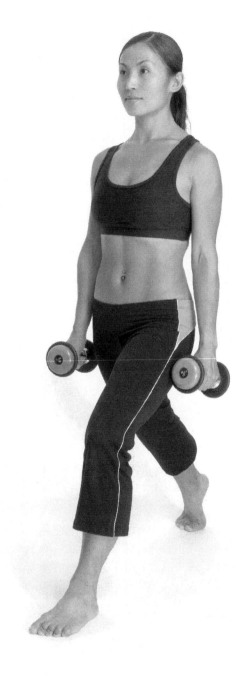

Lunge

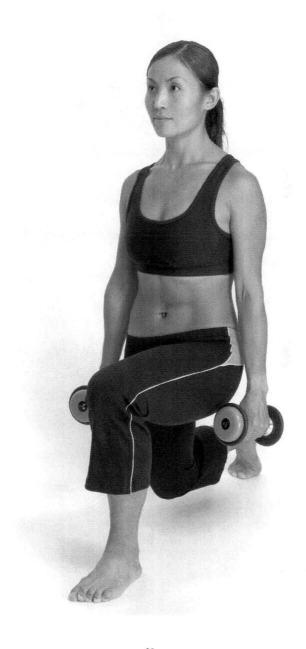

Bent-Over Row

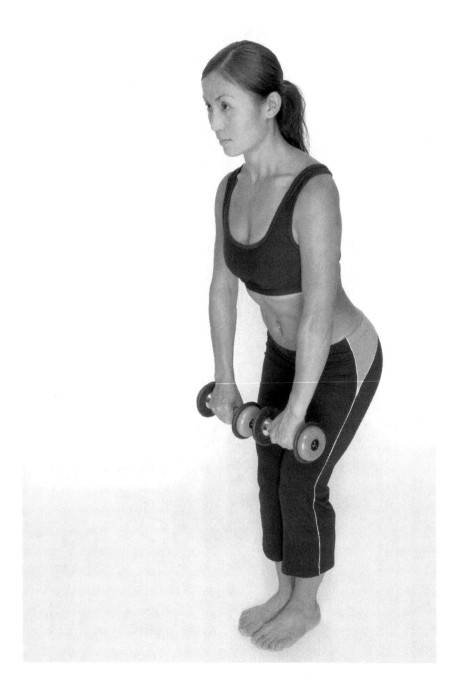

Bent-Over Row

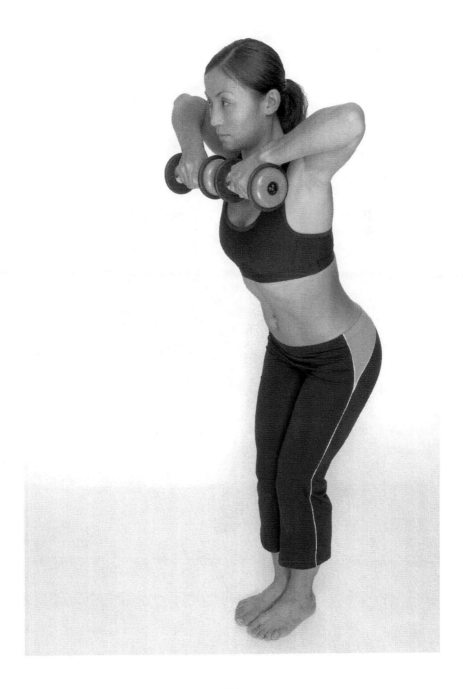

Tricep Extension

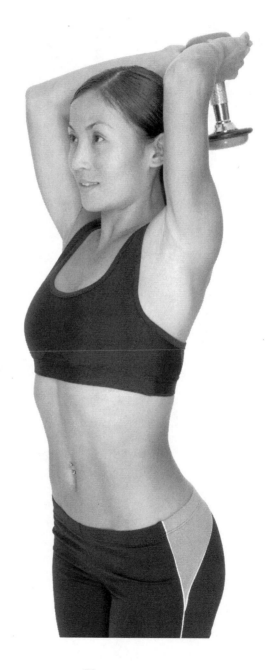

Tricep Extension

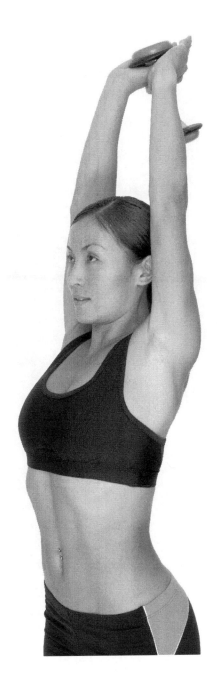

Tricep Kickback

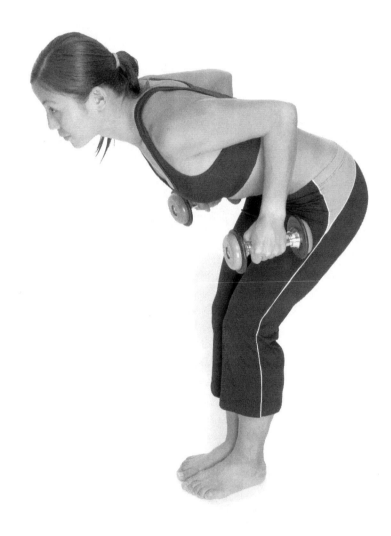

Tricep Kickback

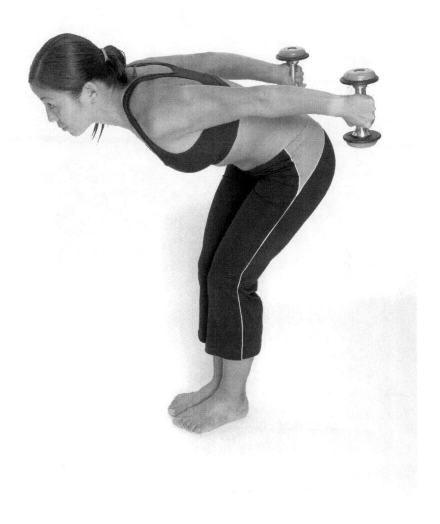

Abdominal Crunch

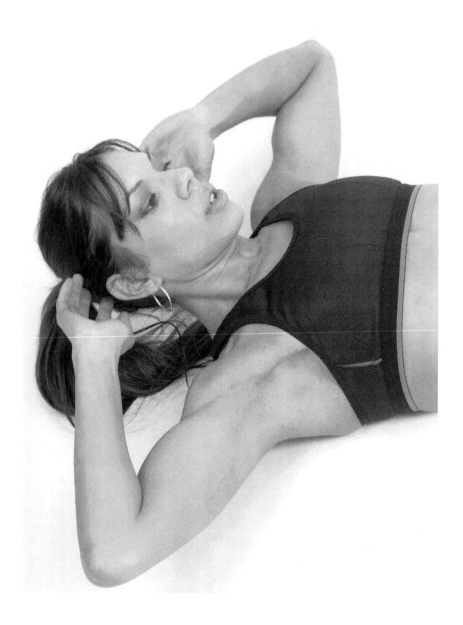

Abdominal Crunch

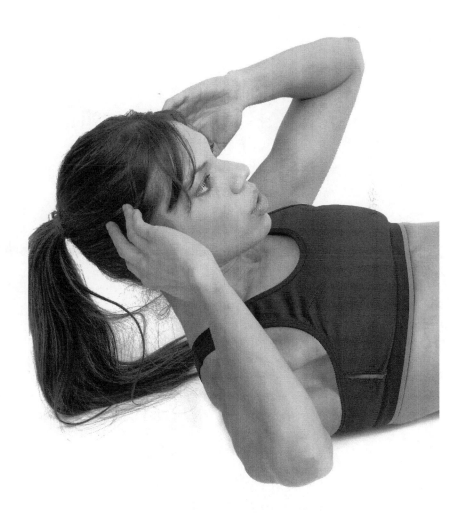

Reversed Abdominal Crunch

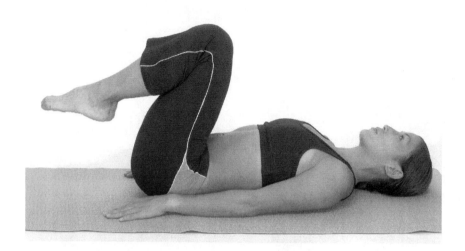

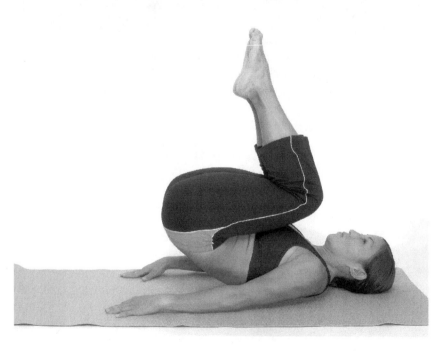

Fly

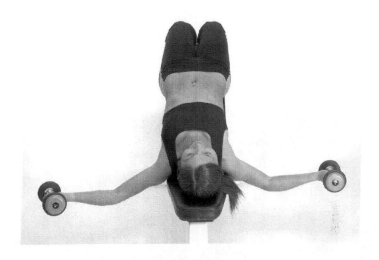

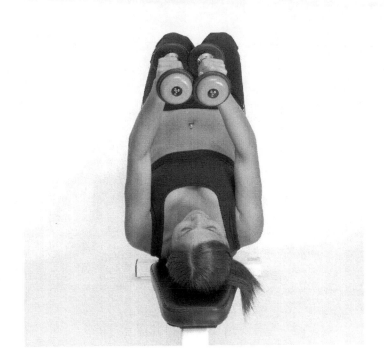

Leg Lift

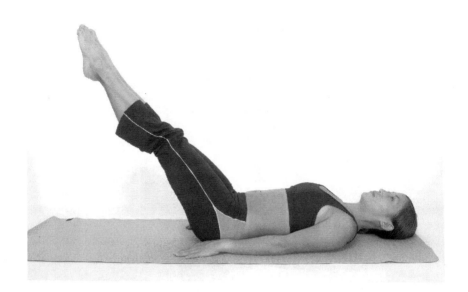

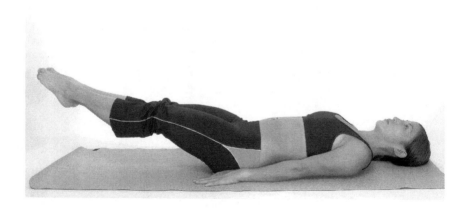

Leg Curl

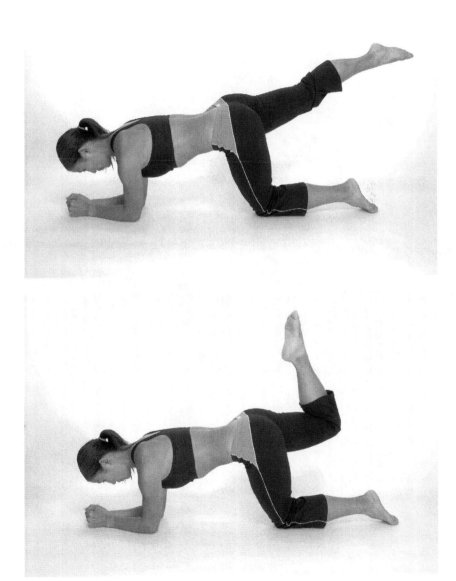

Push-Up

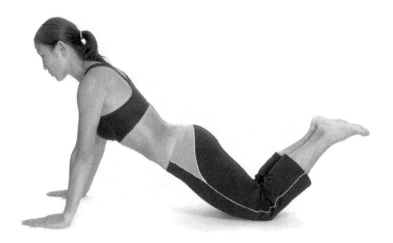

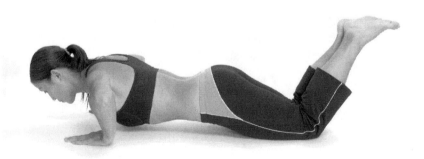

STRETCHES

Stretching is a very important part of the workout routine and is easily overlooked. For optimum performance and flexibility, take the time to stretch before, during, and after each workout and on the days that resistance training is not performed.

Bridge pose

Hip stretch

Back stretch

Hamstrings stretch

Shoulder stretch

Tricep stretch

Side stretch

Shoulder stretch

Chest stretch

Plank pose

Bridge Pose

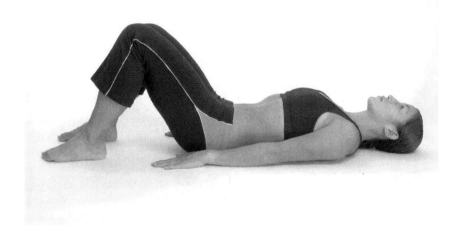

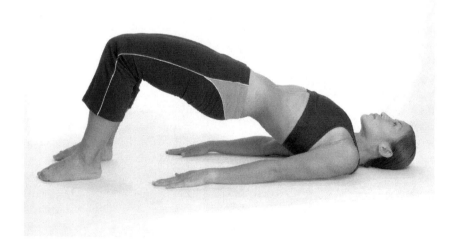

Hip Stretch

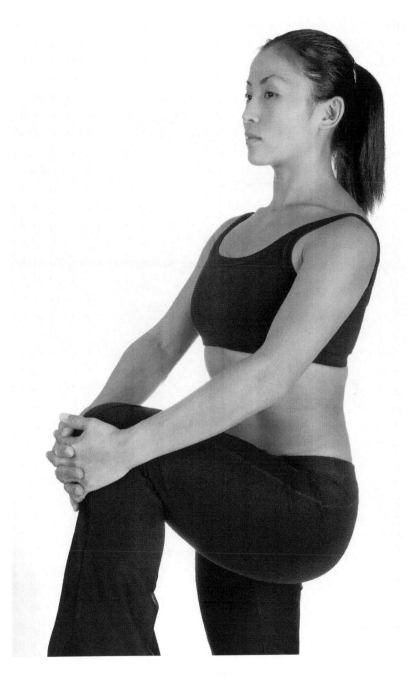

Back Stretch

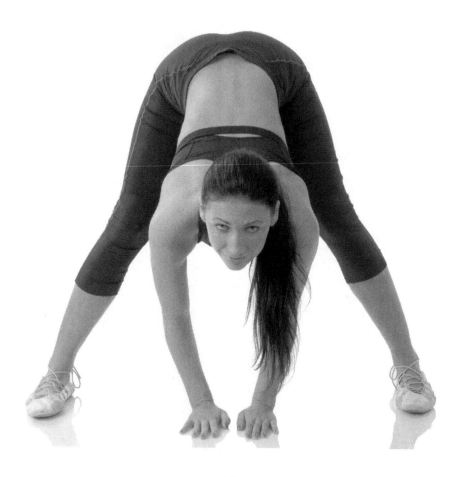

Hamstrings Stretch

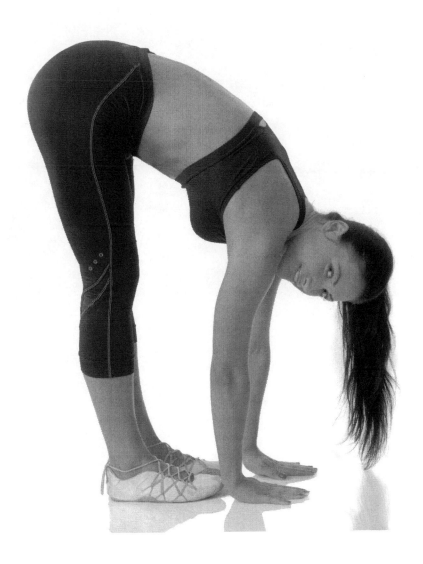

Shoulder Stretch

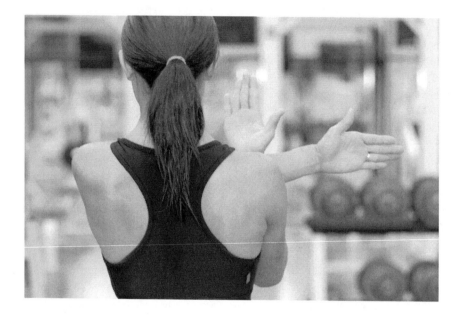

Tricep Stretch

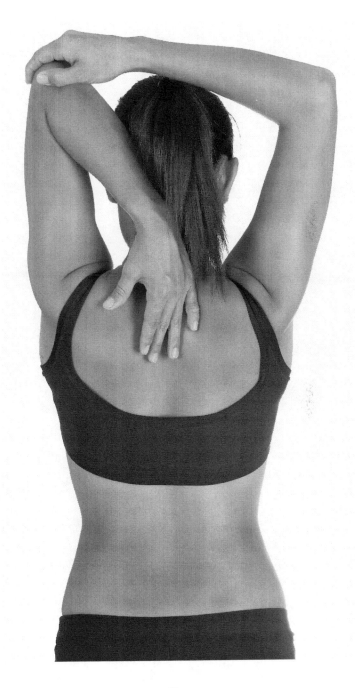

Side Stretch

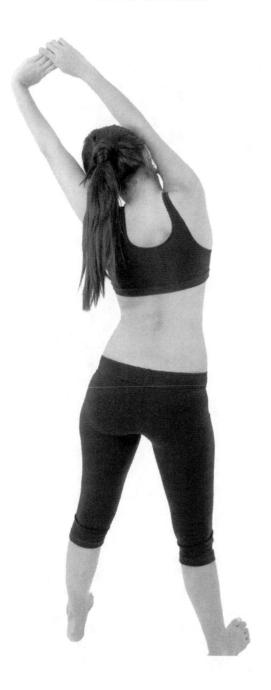

Shoulder Stretch

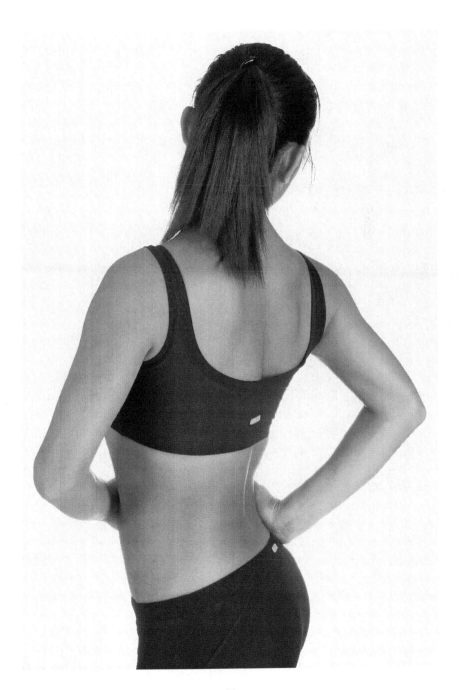

Chest Stretch

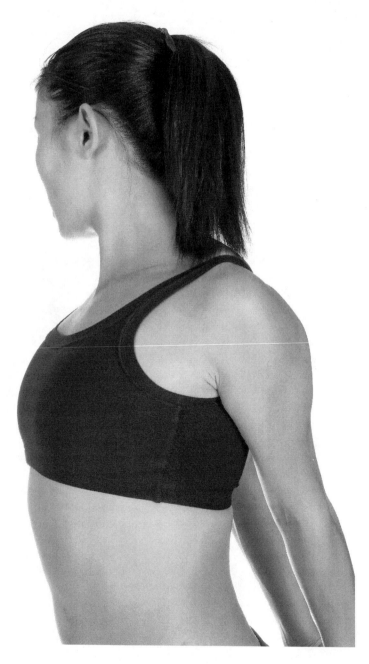

Plank Pose

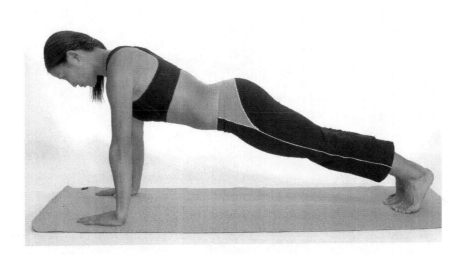

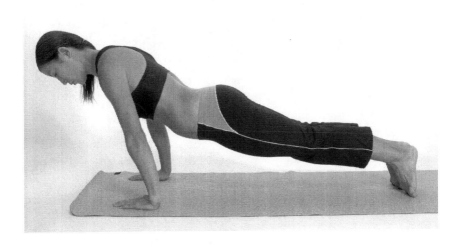

About the Author

Growing up, I was an active child. We lived in the country on a lake, I rode my bike all the time, and we always had a swimming pool. As soon as I reached puberty, I started to notice more fat appearing over my chest and stomach. Several years later, I noticed fat appearing on my upper arms. Over time, the fat increased all over my body, and I became less active. I was uncomfortable and lived with some kind of pain almost daily.

I worked in health care most of my life, and observed firsthand the risks that being over fat can cause. I watched my father suffer with heart disease due to improper healthy nourishment choices, lack of consistent exercise, and smoking.

After many failed attempts for a fast, easy way to lose fat including fad diets and diet supplements, I contemplated different augmentation or weight/fat loss surgeries, but luckily I have a low pain tolerance and chickened out every time especially after I've taken care of numerous patients whose initial surgery turned into a nightmare due to complications, infection, weight bearing on a particular muscle or joint, scar tissue, and multiple surgeries.

I noticed that many health care employees are fat and unhealthy just like me, and we were increasing our own risks of becoming the patient instead of the caregiver.

For years, I tried to incorporated healthy nourishment choices daily prepare meals at home and decrease the number of times that I went out to eat or had fast-food items. I had a multi-gym for a long time, many years later I purchased a resort-size treadmill. For two years, I power walked three or more times a week and covered approximately five to ten miles a week. Because I was burning calories, I lost a couple inches and some weight, but I still had fatty deposits. The more I worked out, the easier it became to make these changes but I felt exhausted after this type of work out and not energized. I remember how I loved feeling strong when I tried to resistance train and I had the multi-station gym at my disposal in addition to several free weight/ dumbbells.

I realized that some of the foods I thought were healthy were actually sabotaging my efforts because of high glycemic index values. I finally learned the importance of these values and how it relates to the nourishment choices that we make every day.

After five years of completing almost eighteen thousand pre op surgery interviews (approx four thousand a year) for anesthesia at an Orthopaedic surgery center, I noticed that the majority of patients are uneducated about their own health.

In my book "Black Jack" to lose fat I discuss the importance that fitness and nutrition have on the body, and I incorporate a program that includes proper nourishment choices to fuel the body and provide energy everyday. It also includes "Black Jack" 21, twenty-one resistance training exercises that will produce lean muscle mass and burn fat. This resistance will be different for each individual and it will depend on the strength of the muscle or joint that is used.

This combination has stabilized my hormones and my mood and blood sugar levels, which has decreased my cravings and desire to binge. It has also decreased my aches and pains and has allowed me to lose the fatty deposits, decreasing my risk for health problems and increasing my life span. In less than a year, I have transformed my physique; the fat literally melted off and still is gone, and I am several sizes smaller than when I began. I am strong! I feel great! My hair, skin, nails, and teeth are in better health than ever before, and others tell me that I look ten years younger.

I encourage anyone who has ever tried to lose fat to take the "Black Jack" to Lose Fat challenge and get *your* body and groove back! And I commend anyone who can shake a weight for one minute, not to mention six minutes!